ESSENTIAL OIL RECIPES

Discover the ultimate collection of DIY aromatherapy blends that will elevate your body, enhance your health, transform your home, and bring harmony to your family.

Dr. Amalie Kleist

Table of Contents

DISCLAIMER

This content is not meant to offer medical advice or replace advice or treatment from a personal physician. It is recommended that you get advice from your doctors or trained health specialists for any specific health inquiries you may have. Readers or followers of this instructional resource are responsible for any potential health effects.

Introduction

Amidst a society saturated with man-made cures and manufactured scents lies a timeless repository of organic marvels eagerly awaiting exploration—the domain of essential oils. Dr. Amalie Kleist's book, "Essential Oil Recipes," offers a captivating exploration of the fragrant realm of holistic well-being and beauty. Dr. Kleist, an esteemed authority in the realm of aromatherapy, cordially welcomes you to dive into the profound wisdom of ancient healing traditions and contemporary scientific investigations, all encapsulated in the concentrated essence of nature's most powerful botanical substances.

Utilizing her extensive expertise and passion for holistic wellbeing, she presents an in-depth guide that enables you to harness the profound potential of essential oils in all facets of your existence.

The core of "Essential Oil Recipes" is a profound respect

for the curative wisdom that plants possess. Dr. Kleist provides valuable information on the medicinal qualities of every essential oil, offering guidance to help you explore and take care of yourself. If you are looking for ways to alleviate stress and anxiety, treat physical diseases, or enhance your beauty, you will discover a variety of recipes specifically designed to meet your individual requirements. This collection meticulously crafts each recipe with a harmonious blend of fragrant lavender and invigorating peppermint, designed to nourish and rejuvenate your physical, mental, and spiritual well-being. Dr. Kleist's recipes are both enjoyable to make and highly successful in producing desired outcomes, whether you are creating an exquisite massage oil, formulating a revitalizing skin serum, or filling your house with a calming fragrance.

However, "Essential Oil Recipes" goes beyond being a mere compilation of mixes. It offers a comprehensive approach to well-being that acknowledges the interdependence of all facets of health. Dr. Kleist imparts her expertise on practicing mindfulness, instructing you on how to develop routines that nourish your inner self and bring balance to your life. By engaging in meditation, breathwork, and easy daily routines, you will acquire the ability to strengthen your bond with nature and activate your inherent capacity for healing.

"Essential Oil Recipes" provides a haven of tranquility and personal well-being in a frequently stressful and daunting environment. This serves as a reminder that even in the middle of the fast-paced and busy nature of contemporary life, the therapeutic influence of nature is readily there, waiting to provide solace, elevate one's spirits, and ignite inspiration.

"Essential Oil Recipes" is a reliable resource for both experienced aromatherapists and those who are new to the practice. It serves as a valuable guide for achieving overall well-being and enhancing attractiveness through the use of essential oils. Allow Dr. Amalie Kleist to serve as your mentor as you begin on a voyage of self-exploration, personal growth, and vibrant well-being. Prepare for an enticing sensory journey.

Chapter One

What are essential oils?

Essential oils are organic, fragrant molecules that occur naturally in different plant components, such as flowers, leaves, stems, roots, and fruits. Usually, they are obtained via distillation or cold pressing, which allows for the capture of the plant's aroma, taste, and advantageous characteristics. We mix the aromatic compounds with a carrier oil after extraction to create a finished product that is ready for use right away.

The method of oil production is crucial because chemically derived essential oils are not considered authentic.

Throughout history, different societies have utilized these oils for their healing, curative, and fragrant properties.

Essential oils are extremely concentrated and powerful, encapsulating the fundamental qualities of the plant they originate from.

How do the components of essential oils function?

Aromatherapists mostly use essential oils, typically inhaling them using a variety of techniques.Ingesting essential oils is not recommended. Essential oils contain compounds that might have various interactions with your body. Some phytochemicals absorb into the skin after topical application.

It is believed that specific techniques of applying a substance can enhance its absorption, such as using heat or applying it to different regions of the body.

Nevertheless, there is a dearth of study in this particular

field. When you breathe in the scents of essential oils, it can activate certain regions of your limbic system. The limbic system is a component of your brain that is involved in emotions, behaviors, sense of smell, and long-term memory. Notably, the limbic system plays a significant role in the formation of memories. This phenomenon can be partially elucidated by the fact that familiar odors have the ability to evoke memories or elicit emotional responses. The limbic system also regulates various involuntary physiological functions, including respiration, cardiac rhythm, and arterial pressure. Therefore, certain individuals argue that essential oils have the ability to produce a tangible impact on your body.

Common varieties

Below is a compilation of 10 widely used essential oils and the corresponding health benefits attributed to them:

- **Peppermint:** it is utilized to enhance energy levels and facilitate the process of digestion.

- **Lavender:** People commonly use it for its ability to reduce tension.

- **Sandalwood:** People use it for its calming qualities and its capacity to improve concentration.

- **Bergamot:** People use it to reduce stress and improve skin conditions like eczema.

- **Rose:** It is utilized for enhancing mood and alleviating anxiety.

- **Chamomile:** It improves mood and promotes relaxation.

- **Ylang-Ylang:** People use it to treat headaches, nausea, and skin problems.

- **Tea Tree:** It is employed to combat infections and enhance immune function.

- **Jasmine:** It is known for its therapeutic effects on

depression, childbirth, and libido.

- **Lemon:** People use it for its beneficial effects on digestion, mood enhancement, headache relief, and other purposes.

Chapter Two

Basic methods for combining essential oils

Basic essential oil mixing techniques involve combining various essential oils to create unique mixes with specific fragrances and medicinal advantages. Here are some basic methods to get you going:

Understanding Notes: We commonly divide essential oils into three primary "notes" based on their rates of evaporation: base, middle, and top notes.

- *Top notes:* There is an instantaneous, bright, and uplifting scent to these oils. They are typically made from herbs or citrus fruits. Peppermint, bergamot, and lemon are a few examples.
- *Middle notes:* Also known as heart notes, these oils provide the blend's substance and contribute to its

overall balance. Usually, they smell vegetal or fragrant. Lavender, geranium, and rosemary are a few examples.

- **Base notes:** These oils have a deep, calming scent that builds slowly and helps to ground the mix. They frequently originate from wood, resins, or roots. Sandalwood, patchouli, and cedarwood are a few examples.

Blending Ratios: It's important to take each essential oil's ratio into account when making a blend. A typical starting point is the following ratio:

- Top notes: 20–30%

- Middle notes: 50–70%

- Base notes: 15–30%

Adjust these percentages depending on your taste and the desired level of intensity for each note in the finished blend.

Layering: Fill the blending container with the base notes first, then the middle notes, and lastly the top notes. This layering method contributes to the harmonic and well-balanced aroma of each oil.

Testing: Prior to producing a larger batch, always test your blend. To test the perfume, place a drop of the mixture on a cotton ball or scent strip and inhale. Applying a small amount (dilution appropriate) to your skin can also be used to monitor for possible skin reactions.

Labeling: After creating a mix, be sure to record the names and ratios of the essential oils used. This will ensure proper usage and help you reproduce the blend in the future.

Experimentation: To make distinctive blends, don't be scared to try out various essential oil combinations. To learn from your mistakes and improve your blending abilities over time, keep a record of your recipes and notes.

Always use pure, premium essential oils and follow usage and dilution safety instructions. You can create your own distinctive mixes that are customized to your tastes and requirements with a little expertise and testing.

The benefits of essential oils

Essential oils have the potential to be utilized in aromatherapy, which is a form of complementary medicine that harnesses the power of scent to enhance one's well-being. Furthermore, one can directly apply these oils to the skin.

Research has shown that essential oils can potentially assist with:

- Enhance the emotional state.
- Improve job performance by minimizing stress levels and increasing focus and alertness.
- Enhance sleep quality.

- Eradicate bacteria, fungi, and viruses.

- Alleviate anxiety and mitigate pain.

- Minimize inflammation.

- Alleviate or diminish feelings of nausea.

- Alleviate migraines.

Essential oils are commonly used for the following purposes:

Aromatherapy: Aromatherapy frequently uses essential oils to encourage calmness, lessen tension, elevate mood, and improve general wellbeing. Breathing in the vapors of essential oils can directly impact the limbic system of the brain, which is responsible for emotions and memory.

Cleaning and household uses: Some essential oils are natural antimicrobials and disinfectants that work well in place of manufactured cleaning supplies. You can use them to clean surfaces, repel pests, and revitalize the air.

Health and wellness: The antibacterial, anti-inflammatory, and antioxidant qualities of many essential oils make them advantageous for promoting physical health. You can apply them topically, take them internally (in certain situations and with caution), or use them aromatically to treat a variety of health ailments, such as pain management, immune system support, digestive troubles, and respiratory troubles.

Skincare: Skincare products frequently include essential oils due to their capacity to nourish and revitalize the skin. When correctly diluted and administered, they can aid in the treatment of acne, aging skin, dryness, inflammation, and other skin disorders.

Although essential oils offer numerous potential benefits, their high concentration necessitates their sparing use. Many times, dilution is required, particularly when administering oils topically, as certain oils might irritate sensitive skin or produce unfavorable reactions. Furthermore, not all essential oils are suitable for internal use, so it's critical to do your homework, use essential oils sensibly, adhere to suggested dosages, and get advice from a licensed healthcare provider as needed.

Guidelines for essential oil dilution

Dilution rules are crucial for the safe and effective use of essential oils, particularly when applying them topically or incorporating them into other DIY recipes. The following are some general recommendations for dilution:

Carrier Oils: Essential oils typically require dilution in a carrier oil before topical application. To help "carry" the essential oils onto the skin and avoid sensitivity or irritation, carrier oils are rich, neutral oils. Jojoba oil, coconut oil, sweet almond oil, and grapeseed oil are examples of common carrier oils.

Ratios of Adult Dilution:

- *General Use:* Adults can safely and effectively use a 2% dilution for the majority of topical applications. This indicates that for every 1 ounce

(30 mL) of carrier oil, add about 12 drops of essential oil.

- *Concentrated Use:* For specific therapies or acute problems, you might use a 5% dilution. This means that for every 1 ounce (30 mL) of carrier oil, there are about 30 drops of essential oil.

For children or people with sensitive skin:

- To lessen the chance of skin irritation, it's best to use a lower dilution ratio on people who have sensitive skin, kids, or the elderly. Typically, experts recommend a 1% dilution for this group, which equates to approximately 6 drops of essential oil per ounce of carrier oil.

Face and Neck: It is recommended to use a lower dilution ratio due to the more fragile nature of the skin in these areas. For facial skincare products, a dilution of 1% to 2% is usually appropriate.

Pregnancy and medical problems: Before using essential oils, anyone who is pregnant, has certain medical problems, or is taking medication should speak with a healthcare provider. Certain oils can interfere with medications or not be safe to use while pregnant.

Patch Test: Apply a tiny amount to a small area of skin and wait 24 hours to check for any adverse responses before applying a diluted essential oil blend over a broad region of the body.

Specific Dilution Recommendations: Dilute certain essential oils in specific ways due to their strength and tendency to cause skin irritation. Certain oils, such as those derived from cinnamon, cloves, and oregano, are deemed "hot" oils and must be well diluted prior to usage.

Always use pure, high-quality essential oils, and heed any particular safety instructions or suggestions given for each oil. Additionally, it's critical to keep essential oils out of children's reach and away from mucous membranes and eyes. If irritation develops, stop using the product right away and wash the area with a carrier oil rather than water.

Tips and tricks for blending essential oils

Although blending essential oils can be a fun and creative process, it's crucial to proceed carefully because essential oils are strong and should only be used sparingly.

The following advice can help you combine essential oils:

Begin with an objective: Ascertain the blend's intended use. Are you trying to achieve energy, relaxation, concentration, or anything else? Having a specific objective in mind will guide your choice of oils.

Recognize the characteristics of the oils: Learn about the characteristics of each essential oil that you intend to utilize. Certain oils offer relaxing or antibacterial qualities, while others are stimulating or anti-inflammatory. By understanding these qualities, you can create a balanced blend.

Consider the smell: Take note of each oil's unique scent and how well they blend together. Try out several combinations to identify scents that work well together.

Use a carrier oil: essential oils are extremely potent and should not be applied directly to the skin as they may irritate it. Before applying them to the skin, always dilute them with a carrier oil like almond, coconut, or jojoba oil.

Start with little amounts: To get the right aroma while combining oils, start with small amounts and add more gradually. This way, you can modify the mixture without wasting any oil.

Maintain a record of ratios: Write down the proportions of each oil you use in your blends so you can duplicate your preferred mixes later.

Experiment: Don't be scared to try out several oil mixes to see which one(s) works best for you. Blending several oils can provide distinctive and pleasing scents.

Think about the base, middle, and top notes: Just like in perfumery, we can divide essential oils into base, middle, and top notes based on their volatility. Combining oils from every category can result in a fragrance character that is well-rounded.

Let blends mature: Before using your blends, give them a few days to mature. This enables the oils to harmonize with one another and allows the aroma to fully develop.

Label your blends: After you've made a blend, label it with the ingredients and ratios. This facilitates sharing or reproducing the blend with others.

Keep safety in mind: Some essential oils are not suitable for use by children, pregnant women, or animals. Investigate each oil's safety thoroughly before incorporating it into your blends.

Trust your sense of smell: Don't force a blend that doesn't smell right to you. Try several combinations until you discover one that works for you.

You can make attractive and useful essential oil mixes that suit your requirements and tastes by using these pointers and techniques.

Chapter Three

11 Common essential oils and their benefits

EUCALYPTUS OIL

Having eucalyptus essential oil on hand is an excellent idea during the colder months. It helps you breathe easier by widening your nasal passageways, which relieves stuffiness in the nose. (Peppermint oil may also be useful in this regard.) Its antibacterial and anti-inflammatory qualities help it combat the herpes simplex virus and reduce discomfort. When using eucalyptus oil, exercise caution and dilute it before applying it topically. It can have harmful adverse effects on children and pets, and it should not be consumed.

LAVENDER OIL

Consider using it as aromatherapy in a bath or diffuser, diluting it with water to create a body spritzer or room spray, or mixing it with a base oil to create body oil.

Lavender is beneficial for pain, stress, and sleep.

Studies have also indicated that the use of tea tree and lavender oils may cause hormonal disruptions in young boys.

FRANKINCENSE OIL

Frankincense, called the "king of oils," is beneficial for mood, sleep, and inflammation. It may also prevent gum disease and help with asthma, according to studies. The woody, spicy perfume of frankincense oil makes it a common ingredient in skin treatments and is also useful in aromatherapy. Before applying frankincense oil to your skin, make sure you dilute it.

ROSEMARY OIL

It's likely that you've reached for rosemary to give some of your recipes more flavor. However, there are also other advantages of taking rosemary oil, such as enhancing mental clarity, encouraging hair development, lowering tension and pain, elevating your mood, and lowering inflammation in your joints. When combined with a carrier oil, rosemary oil is safe to apply directly to the skin and use in aromatherapy. We recommend not using rosemary oil if you have high blood pressure, epilepsy, or are pregnant.

TEA TREE OIL

The majority of individuals use tea tree oil as an antifungal, antiseptic, or antibacterial. It can also be helpful for:

- **Acne.** Dip a cotton swab into the essential oil of the tea tree. After that, put it straight on the acne.
- **Ringworm and athlete's foot.** "Apply the mixture to the afflicted area of skin after diluting it with a

carrier oil, which is a base or vegetable oil like coconut or jojoba oil that helps dilute essential oils."

PEPPERMINT OIL

It is known that peppermint oil:

- Have antibacterial, antifungal, and anti-inflammatory properties.

- Relieve headaches. - Combat exhaustion.

- Uplift your spirits.

- Reduce intestinal spasms.

- Aid in digestion.

- Support memory.

Always dilute the oil before using it topically.

CEDARWOOD OIL

With its pleasant woody aroma, cedarwood oil is a common ingredient in deodorant, shampoo, and insect repellent due to its antioxidant and antibacterial qualities. However, you can also use cedarwood oil to treat anxiety and insomnia.

Cedarwood oil can be applied topically when combined with a carrier oil or used as aromatherapy.

LEMON OIL

Lemon oil is extracted from the peel of lemons and can be applied topically to the skin with a carrier oil or diffused into the atmosphere. The application of lemon oil has demonstrated:

- Lower stress and depression.

- Decrease pain.

- Reduce nausea.

- Eliminate germs.

According to a study, aromatherapy with essential oils, such as lemon oil, may help Alzheimer's patients' cognitive abilities. It is safe to use lemon oil topically as well as for aromatherapy.

However, some reports suggest that applying lemon oil can heighten your skin's susceptibility to sunlight, potentially increasing your risk of sunburn. After using, keep yourself out of the direct sunlight. Lemon, lime, orange, grapefruit, lemongrass, and bergamot oils are among them.

LEMONGRASS OIL

With its potent citrus aroma, lemongrass oil is well-known for its ability to reduce tension, anxiety, and depression. It is an excellent natural medicine for healing wounds and killing infections because of its antibacterial qualities. It has been demonstrated to stop the growth of fungi that cause jock itch, ringworm, and athlete's foot.

A study has shown that lemongrass oil can help people with type 2 diabetes lower their blood sugar levels.

Before applying it to your skin, make sure you use a carrier oil.

ORANGE OIL

Orange oil comes from the rinds of citrus fruits. It can be applied topically to the skin (with a carrier oil), diffused into the air, or even used as a natural cleanser for your home.

Orange oil is recognized to:

- Eliminate germs.

- Decrease anxiety

- Decrease pain.

Applying orange oil to your skin and then stepping outside should be done with caution, as it can cause your skin to become more sensitive to sunlight.

BERGAMOT OIL

You can apply the fruity and floral scent oil topically with a carrier oil or diffuse it (although it may cause photosensitivity).

Bergamot oil is recognized for its ability to:

- Decrease anxiety.

- Improve mood.

- Reduce blood pressure.

Vitality and health-promoting essential oil recipes

There are several ways to use essential oils to support wellbeing and health. Here are several recipes for various uses:

Blend for Immune Support

- Two drops of lemon oil

- Two drops of rosemary oil

- Three drops of eucalyptus oil

- Three drops of tea tree oil

Apply topically to the feet or chest after diluting in a carrier oil and letting the diffuser run for 30 to 60 minutes.

Blends to aid sleep

- Two drops of cedarwood oil

- Three drops of lavender oil

- Two drops of Roman chamomile oil

Apply on the back of the neck and the bottoms of the feet after diluting in carrier oil, or diffuse in the bedroom half an hour before bed.

Never apply essential oils directly to skin without first thoroughly diluting them with a carrier oil. You should also run a patch test to make sure you don't have any sensitivities. Additionally, before taking essential oils, get medical advice if you have any underlying health disorders or concerns.

Muscle-Relaxing Bath Blend

- Five drops of eucalyptus oil

- Five drops of peppermint oil

- Five drops of lavender oil

- Mix with half a cup of Epsom salts and add to a warm bath. Give it a 20–30 minute soak.

Blend for Stress Relief

- Four drops of lavender oil

 - Three drops of chamomile oil

 - Two drops of Frankincense oil

For topical use on pulse points, diffuse in your workspace or dilute in a roller bottle with a carrier oil.

Roll-On for Headache Relief

- Three drops of lavender oil

- Two drops of eucalyptus oil

- Five drops of peppermint oil

Blend using a roller bottle and a carrier oil such as fractionated coconut oil or jojoba oil, then apply to the back of the neck, forehead, and temples.

Blend to Boost Energy

- Two drops of lemon oil

- Three drops of grapefruit oil

- Two drops of peppermint oil

Diffuse in the morning or dilute in a roller bottle for an energizing aroma while on the go.

Chapter Four

10 DIY Essential oil recipes for skin care

To keep your skin looking and feeling good, you must take care of it. The following are some key recipes for natural skin care products:

Oatmeal and Honey Face Mask

Ingredients:

- 1 tablespoon of honey

- 2 teaspoons of oatsmeal.

Instructions: To make a paste, combine the oats and honey. After applying it to your face, rinse it off with warm water after 15 to 20 minutes. Oatmeal calms and exfoliates skin, while honey contains antibacterial qualities and hydrates it.

Essential Oil Roll-On for Acne

Tea tree and oregano, two potent essential oils, work together to help ward off zits before they have a chance to settle in. Apply immediately to the blemishes for healthier, more radiant skin, up to twice a day.

Ingredients:

- 10 ml roll-on bottle

- Grapeseed carrier oil

- 1 drop of oregano essential oil

- 2 drops of Tea Tree Essential Oil

Instructions: To get clear, healthy skin, fill the roll-on bottle with Grapeseed Carrier Oil, add the essential oils, and apply directly to blemishes 1-2 times per day.

Yogurt and Avocado Face Mask

Ingredients:

- ½ ripe avocado

- 1 tablespoon of plain yogurt.

Instructions: Mash the avocado and combine it with the yogurt to create a paste that is smooth. After applying the mask to your face, rinse it off with warm water and let it sit for 15 to 20 minutes. Yogurt has lactic acid, which helps to exfoliate and brighten the skin, while avocado is full of vitamins and fatty acids that feed the skin.

Sugar Scrub with Coconut Oil

Ingredients:

- 1 tablespoon sugar (brown or white)

- 2 tablespoons of coconut oil.

Instructions: Combine sugar and coconut oil to make a scrub. Use circular motions to gently massage the scrub onto your skin. Rinse with warm water. Sugar exfoliates the skin and contains antibacterial and hydrating qualities for the skin.

Rosehip with Lemon Oil Face Mask for Acne

Ingredients:

- 1/3 cup of unrefined honey

- 1/3 cup plain yogurt

- 2 tablespoons of rosehip oil

- Drops of lemon oil

Instructions: Combine all the ingredients in a small container and cover it. Mix everything well. After applying, leave it on your face for about 10 minutes. After removing it with a washcloth and warm water, gently wipe the skin dry.

Rosewater and Witch Hazel Toner

Ingredients:

- 1/2 cup of rosewater

- 1/4 cup witch hazel.

Directions: Combine the witch hazel and rosewater. After cleansing, apply the mixture to your skin using a cotton ball or pad. Witch hazel is a natural astringent that can help to tighten pores and lessen irritation, while rosewater contains anti-inflammatory qualities and hydrates the skin.

Honey and Turmeric Face Mask

Ingredients:

- 1 tsp. powdered turmeric

- 1 tablespoon of honey

- 1 tsp. yogurt (may be skipped).

Instructions: To make a paste, combine the yogurt, honey, and turmeric powder. After applying the mask to your face, rinse it off with warm water and let it sit for ten to fifteen minutes. Honey soothes and hydrates, while turmeric's antimicrobial and anti-inflammatory qualities can help minimize acne and brighten the skin.

Jojoba with Lavender Oil Foot Dip

This foot dip recipe employs Epsom salts to treat tired feet while inducing deep relaxation throughout the body via the soles of the feet. Lavender oil brings calm, and geranium oil balances. After only 10 minutes of this calming, DIY foot dip, you'll feel incredibly calm. Ingredients:

- 1 cup of baking soda

- 1/4 cup of Epsom salts

- 1 teaspoon jojoba oil

- 5 drops of lavender essential oil

- 5 drops of Geranium Rose Oil

Instructions: Mix every component together and transfer around 1/4 into a small bathtub that has warm water in it. Give your feet a 15-minute soak.

Green Tea Toner

Ingredients:

- 1 cup of cool, brewed green tea

- 1 tablespoon vinegar made from apple cider (optional).

Instructions: Stir the apple cider vinegar (if using) into the green tea. After cleansing, apply the mixture to your skin using a cotton ball or pad. While apple cider vinegar helps to balance pH levels, green tea, which is high in antioxidants, can help soothe and tone the skin.

Banana Lemon with Essential Oil Cleanser

When combined with almond oil, bananas are a fantastic natural skincare ingredient that provides intense moisture.

Ingredients:

- 1 ripe, mashed banana

- A squeeze of fresh lemon juice

- 1/2 teaspoon almond oil

- 2 drops carrot oil 2 drops of Neroli Oil

Instructions: Mix the ingredients in a bowl and apply the mixture, avoiding the eyes, to your forehead, nose, chin, and cheeks. Give the cleanser a few minutes to work its magic. With a fresh washcloth and warm water, remove.

Never forget to conduct a patch test on your face before applying any new components, particularly if you have sensitive skin. Additionally, before experimenting with new skincare recipes, see a dermatologist if you have any sensitivities or skin issues.

Essential oils can help with eight skin issues.

1. Reduce Pore Size

If you possess enlarged or obstructed pores, it is imperative to take action in order to reduce their size and prevent blockage.

Tea tree oil can address both issues.

After dilution, gently apply and rub the substance onto your facial skin for approximately five minutes. Thoroughly wash and gently dry by patting.

2. Enhance the firmness of your skin.

There are numerous options of oils available for you to experiment with in order to enhance the firmness of your skin.

Loose skin is a common occurrence as one ages, however, it can be mitigated by using frankincense and/or lavender essential oil.

3. Decelerate the process of aging.

By utilizing appropriate essential oils, you can contribute to the deceleration of the aging process and maintain the health and radiance of your skin.

Consider experimenting with unconventional remedies such as carrot seed oil, known for its efficacy in counteracting sun-induced skin damage.

4. Maintain Balance with Oily Skin

Individuals with oily skin typically experience pimples as well.

Firstly, it is important to comprehend that possessing oily skin is not inherently negative, as it tends to decelerate the aging process of our skin.

The key is to maintain the cleanliness of your pores.

Consider utilizing tea tree oil, ylang-ylang, and chamomile essential oil if you have sensitive skin.

5. Relieve skin dryness.

Individuals with dry skin may be susceptible to experiencing itching and developing rashes.To alleviate dry skin, essential oils are the solution.

Experiment with combinations of frankincense, sandalwood, sage, and rose in jojoba oil.

6. Combat acne

Tea tree, peppermint, and eucalyptus oils possess beneficial properties for combating acne, as do citrus oils.

7. Minimize the formation of scars.

If you have a tendency to develop scars easily or if you already have scars from acne, it may be beneficial for you to incorporate carrot seed oil, citrus oils, and vitamin E oil into your skincare routine.

8. Enhance the condition of eczema.

If you have this ailment, you are aware that it is a perpetual struggle, and it is not always possible to pinpoint the trigger for a sudden worsening of symptoms.

Chapter Five

15 DIY Essential oil recipes for home care

Organic Carpet Deodorizer

Ingredients

1 cup of sodium bicarbonate

15 droplets of lavender essential oil

10 drops of lemon essential oil

5 drops of tea tree essential oil.

Directions: Combine all ingredients in a jar and mix well. Disperse evenly onto carpets, allow to remain for 15-20 minutes, then thoroughly remove with a vacuum.

Antimicrobial Hand Sanitizer

Ingredients

2/3 cup of isopropyl alcohol (with a minimum concentration of 70%)

1/3 cup aloe vera gel

10 drops of tea tree essential oil

10 drops of lavender essential oil

Instructions: Mix all ingredients in a bowl until well combined. Transfer the contents to a small container for convenient application.

Natural Dish Soap

Ingredients

1 cup of liquid castile soap

2 teaspoons of white vinegar

10 droplets of lemon essential oil

5 droplets of orange essential oil

Directions: Pour all ingredients into a bottle that has a flip-top cap. Utilize this product in the same manner as you would conventional dish soap.

Odor-neutralizing aerosol

Ingredients

1 cup of distilled water

2 teaspoons of vodka or rubbing alcohol

10 droplets of eucalyptus essential oil

10 drops of peppermint essential oil

5 droplets of lemon essential oil

Directions: Mix together all the ingredients in a spray container and vigorously shake until fully blended. Utilize this product to invigorate and cleanse various spaces, such as rooms, closets, or upholstery.

Essential Oil-Based Floor Cleaner

Ingredients

¼ cup grated castile soap

¼ cup white vinegar

25–30 drops of a vital oil, particularly lemon-scented

1 gallon of hot water

Directions: Combine vinegar and castile soap, then incorporate essential oil. Take a bucket filled with hot water and add the homemade floor cleaner. Stir the mixture thoroughly. Utilize a mop to thoroughly cleanse your floor using the provided solution.

Essential Oil Wood Floor Cleaner

Ingredients

1 gallon of water at a comfortably high temperature

1/2 cup white vinegar

10 droplets of pine essential oil

5 drops of lemon essential oil

Directions: Combine all ingredients in a bucket. Use a mop to clean wood floors, making sure to squeeze out any excess moisture from the mop.

Daily Shower Spray

Ingredients

1 cup of white vinegar

1 cup of water

20 droplets of tea tree essential oil

10 drops of eucalyptus essential oil

Directions: Combine all ingredients in a spray bottle. Following a shower, apply a fine mist to the surfaces of shower walls and curtains to inhibit the growth of mold and mildew.

Multi-purpose cleaner

Ingredients

2 cups of distilled water

1/2 cup of white vinegar

10 drops of tea tree essential oil

10 drops of lemon essential oil

5 droplets of lavender essential oil

Directions: Combine all components in a spray container. Agitate well prior to each application. Apply a fine mist to surfaces, and then use a cloth to remove any dirt or residue.

Air Freshener

Ingredients

1 cup of purified water

2 teaspoons of vodka or rubbing alcohol

10 droplets of your preferred essential oil (such as lavender, peppermint, or citrus)

Directions: Combine the contents in a spray container and vigorously shake to ensure thorough mixing. Disperse a fine mist across the room to improve the air quality.

Natural Fabric Softener

Ingredients

1 cup of white vinegar

1 cup of baking soda

20 droplets of lavender essential oil

Directions: Combine vinegar and essential oil in a container. Gradually incorporate baking soda, as it will produce effervescence. Continuously mix until fully incorporated. For optimal fabric softening, add 1/4 cup of the product per load during the rinse cycle.

Laundry Fragrance Enhancer

Ingredients

1 cup of Epsom salt

15-20 drops of your favorite essential oil

Directions: Combine the Epsom salt and essential oils in a jar. To infuse a pleasant aroma, incorporate 1-2 tablespoons into every laundry cycle prior to washing.

Furniture Polish

Ingredients

1/4 cup olive oil

1/4 cup white vinegar

10 droplets of lemon essential oil

Directions: Combine the ingredients in a small bowl. Take a tiny quantity of the product and apply it to a microfiber cloth. Then, use the cloth to polish wooden furniture.

Insect repellent

Ingredients

1/4 cup witch hazel

1/4 cup of distilled water

20 drops of citronella essential oil

10 droplets of lavender essential oil 10 drops of peppermint essential oil

Directions: Blend all components in a spray container and vigorously agitate. Apply the spray to your skin or clothing prior to stepping outside.

Linen Spray for Sleepy Time

Ingredients

1/2 cup of distilled water

1 tablespoon of either witch hazel or vodka.

10 droplets of lavender essential oil

5 droplets of chamomile essential oil

Directions: Combine the contents in a spray container and vigorously shake until well blended. Apply a gentle mist to pillows and sheets prior to going to sleep.

Antifungal Solution

Ingredients

1 cup of distilled water

1 cup of white vinegar

10 droplets of tea tree essential oil

10 droplets of lemon essential oil

Directions: Combine the contents in a spray container and vigorously shake until well blended. Apply the spray to surfaces that are affected by mold or mildew and allow it to remain for a duration of 10 minutes before cleaning it away.

These recipes provide organic and efficient substitutes for different cleaning requirements within the household. Prior to usage, it is imperative to vigorously shake the product and conduct a preliminary test on a small, inconspicuous region, particularly on fragile surfaces.

Chapter Six

Essential oil recipes for emotional support

There are several ways that essential oils can provide emotional assistance. The following is a list of popular essential oils for emotional support, along with the attributes that go along with each one

LAVENDER: Known for its balancing and calming properties, lavender essential oil helps ease tension, ease anxiety, and promote relaxation.

BERGAMOT: Bergamot essential oil has a citrus aroma that is energizing and helps reduce anxiety and depressive symptoms while elevating mood.

CHAMOMILE (ROMAN): Roman chamomile essential oil is soothing and calming, making it useful for stress management, irritation reduction, and relaxation.

FRANKINCENSE: This grounded, earthy essential oil can aid in emotional healing, lower anxiety levels, and foster inner serenity.

YLANG YLANG: The perfume of fragrant flowers in ylang ylang essential oil can help lower stress, improve mood, and encourage emotions of joy and sensuality.

CLARY SAGE: Known for its uplifting and euphoric properties, clary sage essential oil is helpful in establishing emotional balance, regulating mood swings, and reducing anxiety.

ROSE: The deep, flowery scent of rose essential oil is associated with emotional healing, love, and compassion. It can lift people up and encourage acceptance and self-love.

PATCHOULI: Due to its ability to anchor and balance emotions, patchouli essential oil is helpful in reducing tension and anxiety, as well as fostering a sense of calmness.

SANDALWOOD: The warm, woody scent of sandalwood essential oil helps ease stress and anxiety while fostering calmness and relaxation of the mind.

GERANIUM: Geranium essential oil can help reduce stress and anxiety and support emotional stability since it has a balancing influence on emotions.

You can use these essential oils separately or combine them to create customized mixes that offer emotional support. These essential oils can be dispersed, inhaled directly from the bottle, mixed into bathwater, or diluted in a carrier oil for massage or topical treatment. It is crucial to utilize essential oils in a safe manner and consistently conduct a patch test prior to placing them on the skin. Prior to using essential oils for emotional support, it is advisable to get guidance from a certified aromatherapist or healthcare expert, especially if you have any pre-existing health disorders or concerns.

DIY Essential oil recipes for emotional wellness

Here are some easy DIY essential oil blends for emotional wellness that you can prepare at home:

Calming and Balancing Essential oil Mix

Ingredients:

4 drops of lavender essential oil

3 drops of Bergamot essential oil

2 drops of Roman Chamomile essential oil

1 drop of Frankincense essential oil

1 oz (30 ml) of carrier oil (such as sweet almond oil, jojoba

oil, or coconut oil)

Directions:

- Place the designated quantity of drops of each essential oil into a glass bottle or rollerball that is free of any dirt or impurities.

- Fill the remaining volume of the bottle with your selected carrier oil, ensuring there is a tiny gap at the top to allow for mixing.

- Securely seal the bottle and gently agitate to thoroughly mix the oils.

- Allow the mixture to harmonize for several hours or overnight before using.

Instructions for use:

- Administer just a little of the mixture to your wrists, temples, chest, or nape of the neck to facilitate rapid absorption.

- Inhaling the scent straight from the bottle or by dabbing a few drops onto a cotton ball or handkerchief is another option.

- To create a soothing bathing experience, incorporate a small amount of the mixture into your bathwater and immerse yourself for a duration of 15-20 minutes.

Utilize this mix whenever you have stress, anxiety, or require emotional assistance.

Boosting and Grounding Essential Oil Mix

Ingredients:

4 drops of Bergamot essential oil

3 drops of geranium essential oil

2 drops of cedarwood essential oil

1 drop of Frankincense essential oil

1 oz (30 ml) of jojoba oil (or the carrier oil of your choice)

Directions:

-    Place the required quantity of drops of each essential oil into a clean glass bottle or rollerball.

- Fill the remaining portion of the bottle with jojoba oil, ensuring there is a tiny gap at the top to allow for mixing.

- Securely seal the bottle and gently agitate it to properly combine the oils.

Instructions for use:

- Administer a modest quantity of the mixture to your wrists, temples, or the nape of your neck whenever you require assistance with your emotions or a sense of stability.

- Alternatively, you may inhale the fragrance directly from the bottle or introduce a small quantity into a diffuser.

- To provide a soothing massage, dilute the mixture even further in carrier oil and apply it to your skin through massage.

- Utilize this mix when engaging in meditation, yoga, or at any moment when you desire to cultivate a feeling of balance and elevation.

Bergamot and geranium essential oils have renowned boosting qualities, aiding in the elevation of mood and the alleviation of tension and anxiety. Cedarwood offers a sense of stability and grounding, while frankincense contributes to a feeling of calmness and spiritual grounding. Jojoba oil functions as a nourishing carrier oil, providing gentle hydration to the skin while facilitating the proper absorption of essential oils.

Stress-Soothing Relief Essential Oil Mix

Ingredients:

4 drops of lavender essential oil

3 drops of Roman Chamomile essential oil

2 drops of Frankincense essential oil

1 drop of Ylang Ylang essential oil1 oz (30 ml) fractionated coconut oil (or your preferred carrier oil)

Directions:

- Place the designated quantity of drops of each essential oil into a glass bottle or rollerball that is free from dirt or impurities.

- Complete the remaining portion of the bottle with fractionated coconut oil, ensuring there is a tiny gap at the top to allow for mixing.

- Securely seal the bottle and gently agitate to properly combine the oils.

Instructions for use:

- Administer a modest quantity of the mixture to your

areas of high blood flow, such as the wrists, temples, or behind the ears, whenever you experience feelings of tension or anxiety.

- You can also inhale the relaxing scent directly from the container or add a few drops to a diffuser.

- To achieve a soothing massage, dilute the mixture more in carrier oil and apply it to your neck, shoulders, or any other areas of tension.

Utilize this mix prior to going to bed to facilitate relaxation and enhance the quality of sleep.

Lavender essential oil is renowned for its soothing and tranquilizing qualities, which aid in stress reduction and the promotion of a serene state of mind. Roman chamomile further promotes relaxation and alleviates nervous tension. Frankincense offers a sense of stability and reduces anxiety, while Ylang Ylang contributes a pleasant floral fragrance that enhances mood and fosters emotional equilibrium.

Alcohol Addiction Quitting Essential Oil Mix

Ingredients:

8 ml of sweet almond oil

4 drops of lemon essential oil

4 drops of ginger essential oil

4 drops of lavender essential oil

4 drops of rosemary essential oil

4 drops of peppermint essential oil

Directions:

- Transfer each essential oil individually into a 10 ml glass container, ensuring to blend thoroughly after adding each one.

- Once you've thoroughly mixed the ingredients, add sweet almond oil or any other carrier oil of your choice.

- Ensure that you allocate sufficient space.

- Open the cover and vigorously agitate it.

- You can now employ your essential oil blend to address alcoholism.

Instructions for use

You can utilize essential oils in various ways to benefit from their diverse range of properties

- Breathe in the aromatic compounds of the essential oils.

- Topical use (Not recommended for very concentrated oils)

- Aromatic baths with essential oils should be complemented with the use of Epsom salt.

Essential Oil Mix for Sleep and

Relaxation

Ingredients:

3 drops of lavender essential oil

2 drops of Roman Chamomile essential oil

2 drops of Cedarwood essential oil

2 drops of sweet orange essential oil

Directions:

- Prepare your essential oil combination for storage in a clean, dark glass bottle.

- Fill the bottle with the prescribed number of drops of each essential oil.

- Tightly close the bottle and give it a good shake to mix the oils well.

Instructions for use

Diffusion: Prior to going to sleep, incorporate 3-5 droplets of the mixture into your essential oil diffuser. Allow it to disperse throughout your bedroom for around 30 minutes prior to going to sleep.

Pillow Spray: Mix a tiny amount of the blend with water and transfer it to a small spray bottle. Apply a small amount of spritz to your pillow and bedding prior to going to sleep.

Inhale: Apply a small amount of the mixture to a tissue or cotton ball and place it below your pillowcase or in close proximity to your bedside. Breathe in deeply to savor the fragrance as you fall asleep.

Lavender is renowned for its calming and soothing qualities, making it optimal for facilitating relaxation and enhancing sleep quality.

Roman chamomile possesses a mild sedative effect that aids in soothing the mind and body prior to sleep.

Cedarwood possesses an earthy scent that has the ability

to promote a sense of calmness and alleviate stress.The addition of sweet orange oil brings a vibrant and uplifting component to the mixture while also encouraging a state of relaxation.

ACKNOWLEDGEMENTS

All glory belongs to God. I'd also want to thank my wonderful family, partner, fans, readers, friends, and customers for their constant support and words of encouragement.

www.ingramcontent.com/pod-product-compliance
Lightning Source LLC
Chambersburg PA
CBHW031133020426
42333CB00012B/354